Strength Training Workout at Home

The Ultimate Home Workout Plan

Copyright © 2020

All rights reserved.

DEDICATION

Contents

Introduction

Build a brand new body by performing functional exercises with some classic kit – dumbbells

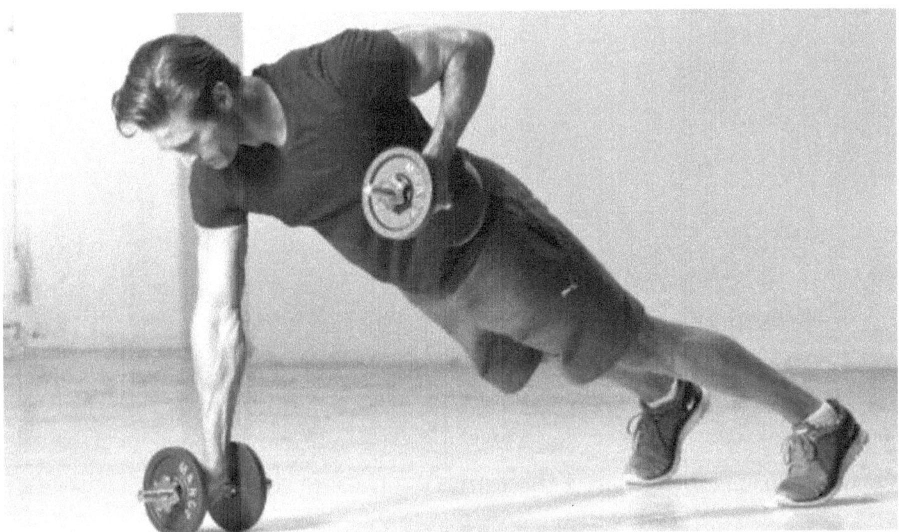

The fitness industry can sometimes seem like a bewildering blur of new ideas, with novel diets, workout classes and equipment cropping up constantly, surrounded by hype that claims they're the best possible way to get fit. If that sort of thing leaves you cold, it should be reassuring to know that it can all be ignored in favour of a far more traditional route to fitness – a set of dumbbells and a few well-planned home workouts.

There's a good chance you already have the dumbbells, sitting around somewhere gathering dust, but if you don't then take a look at our selection of the best dumbbells to find a set that suits you. There are options for all comers, whether you're after the cheapest set you can find – it's just a weight with a handle, after all – or ready to splash out on some durable cast iron, shiny chrome, or some-kind-of-black-magic adjustable dumbbells that change the weight for you at the click of a button.

What are the benefits of strength training?

Research has shown that strength training can benefit your health and fitness in many different ways. According to the Mayo Clinic, strength training may help:

- Build lean muscle mass
- Reduce body fat
- Burn calories more efficiently, even after you've exercised
- Boost metabolism and make weight loss easier
- Increase bone density and improve bone health
- Boost flexibility and improve range of motion
- Improve brain health and cognitive functions
- Reduce the symptoms of many chronic conditions, including back pain, diabetes, arthritis, and heart disease
- Improve posture, balance, and stability
- Raise energy levels
- Improve mood and overall sense of well-being

What are the benefits of working out at home?

- A home-based exercise routine can be a super easy and convenient way of fitting in a workout without having to hit the gym.
- Benefits
- It saves time. There's no traveling or waiting for machines or equipment.
- It's low cost. There are no gym fees or expensive equipment needed.
- Work out anytime. You can exercise on your own schedule, no matter the time of day or night.
- Privacy. You can work out without feeling self-conscious.
- Go at your own pace. There's no pressure to keep up with those around you or to push yourself beyond what's comfortable.

Getting started

Once you're ready to start putting together your strength training workout, the first step is to find a place in your home where you can exercise comfortably. You'll want to find an area that has enough room for you to move your arms and legs freely.

You don't need to invest in much equipment, but if you do want to purchase a few items, here are some that may be helpful:

an exercise mat

resistance bands or tubing

dumbbells

a kettlebell

a stability ball

a medicine ball

Instead of using dumbbells or a kettlebell, you can improvise by using water bottles, sandbags, or canned goods in place of the weights.

If you're just getting started with strength training, you may want to find a strength training workout for beginners online. This can help you learn how to do different exercises with the right form, and also

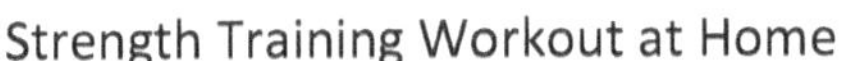

warm up and cool down correctly.

Start with a warmup

Before starting your workout, do a warmup routine for at least 5 to 10 minutes. This can include brisk walking, jogging on the spot, or movements that work your legs, arms, and other major muscle groups.

12 At-Home Workouts You Can Do Without Any Equipment

You can get results with just your bodyweight.

The best at-home workouts don't necessarily require a ton of equipment—or *any* equipment—other than your own bodyweight. That's good news for many exercisers who may not have dumbbells, kettlebells, resistance bands, or other equipment at home, especially after the closures of gyms and fitness studios (and the recommendations to practice social distancing) due to the new coronavirus.

If you don't have a lot of equipment, at-home bodyweight workouts are clutch and allow you to keep up your fitness routine. You might *think* your options are limited if you don't have a whole rack of equipment at your disposal, but that's definitely not the case. You can use bodyweight exercises to work nearly every muscle in your body, from your quads (squats) to your butt (glute bridges, anyone?) to your chest (yes, you *can* do a push-up!) to your core (plank variations for the win!).

They're not just great for building strength, though: Bodyweight workouts can double as a cardio routine, especially when you choose moves that are easy to ramp up in intensity and perform them in such a way—usually circuit-style, with limited rest—that challenges you cardiovascularly.

Plus, there are a *ton* of bodyweight exercises out there, meaning the possibilities for bodyweight workouts are nearly endless, and we've rounded up a bunch of them for you here. Want to really home in on your lower body? Workout #1 may be for you. Looking to get just as sweaty as when you run? Try #6. And if you're looking for a way to strengthen your shoulders and arms, #11 may be one to try.

Whatever your intended goal of the workout, the list below of the best at-home workouts that require only your bodyweight has you covered. Try a bunch of these workouts from SELF to figure out your favorites!

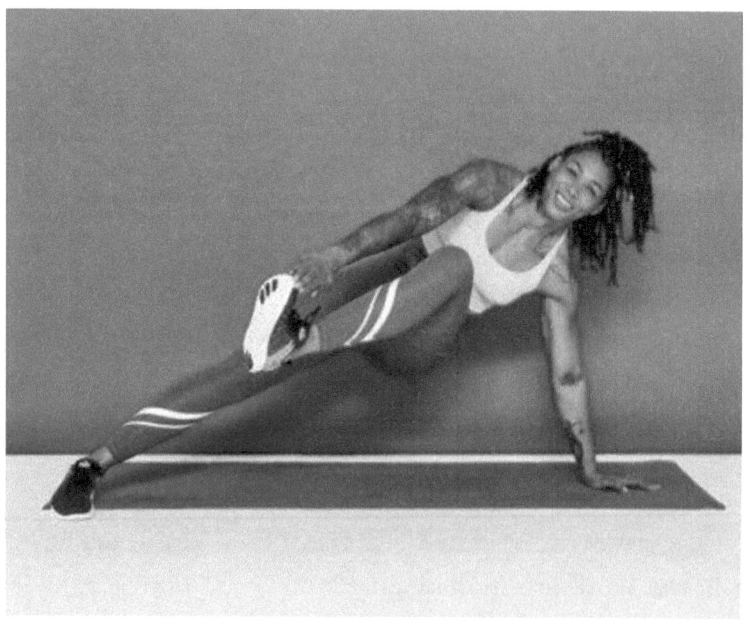

1

A Lower-Body Workout With Cardio Burnout

This isn't your regular old leg workout—there are a few exercises in here that we bet you haven't tried yet, like the runner's-lunge-to-balance (great for speed and agility) and the corkscrew (a dynamic plank variation that'll seriously test your core strength). Created by Amy Eisinger, C.P.T., this workout will test your endurance all the way through. And then just when you think you're done, there's a cardio burnout at the end that'll give you one last challenge. You can make it easier or harder by tweaking the amount of rest you take between exercises in the circuit. Try the workout.

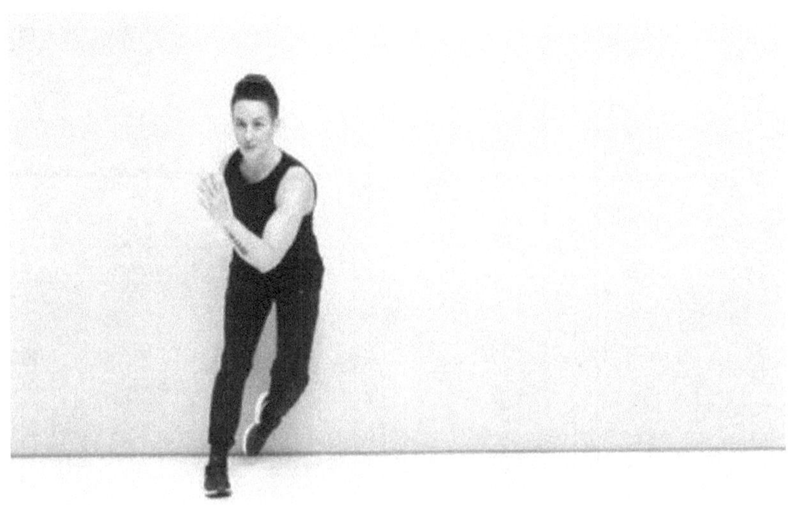

2

A 20-Minute HIIT Workout That's Kinder on Your Joints

Lots of at-home HIIT workouts are chock-full of plyometric moves (read "lots of jumping"), which is great for some people, but not the best choice for those who may have some problems with their joints. This HIIT workout, which was created by Equinox group fitness instructor Colleen Conlon, is kinder on the joints than most HIIT workouts, since it includes lower-impact moves like side kick throughs and crab toe touches. There still are *some* moves that are a little higher impact, like skater hops, so if you're not sure if this workout would be safe for you, talk to your doctor or physical therapist first.

Try the workout.

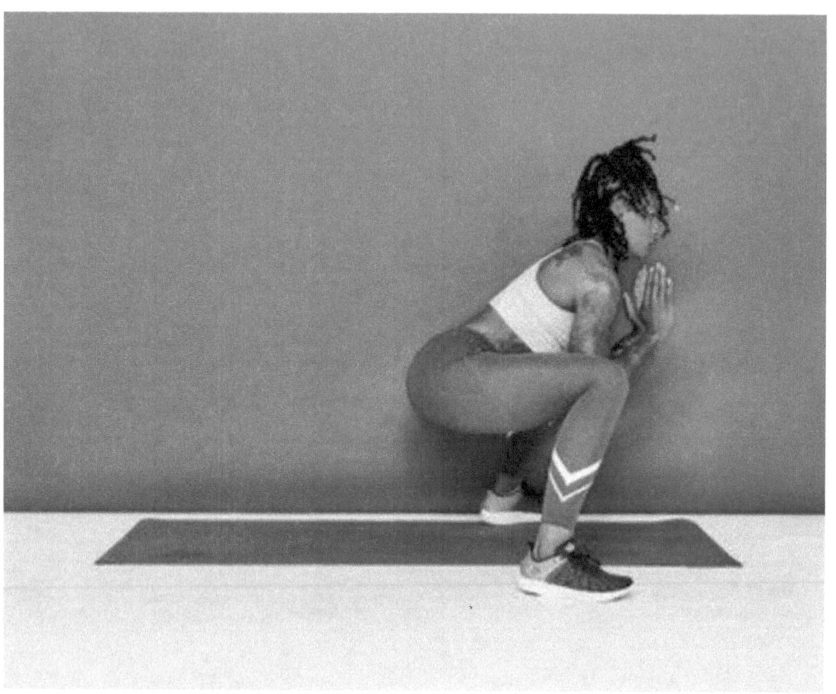

3

A Full-Body Cardio Challenge

Want an at-home cardio workout that works your whole body? Then you'll have to give this routine, created by Eisinger, a try. The circuit will cycle through five moves, which work everything from your legs (squat pulse), core (tuck-up), and shoulders (frogger). Once you complete the circuit for your chosen number of rounds, you'll finish with a AMRAP (as many reps as possible) finisher.

Try the workout.

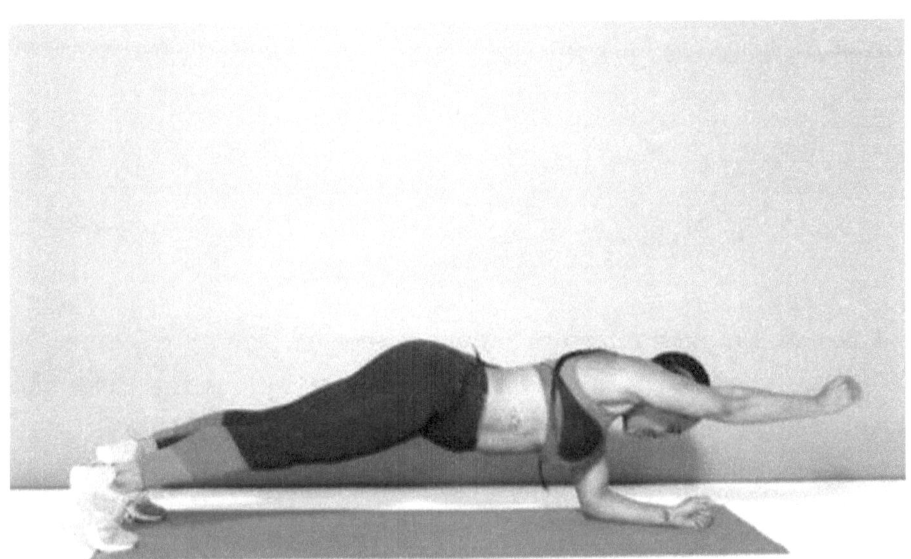

4

A Plank-Based Workout to Light Up Your Core

Yes, you can work your arms with just your bodyweight. And a great way to do that is through variations of the plank, where your shoulders and triceps really put in the work. Created by certified trainer Lita Lewis, this workout will start with skaters to get your blood pumping, and then take you to the floor for the next three plank-based moves: push-up, shoulder tap, and plank forearm reach. The second circuit is heavy on the plank variations too, with the plank jack and forearm plank. You'll be tasked with holding the plank for a good chunk of time with these moves (since they're back-to-back-to-back), so if it's too hard to maintain with good form, drop to your knees to make it a bit easier.

Try the workout.

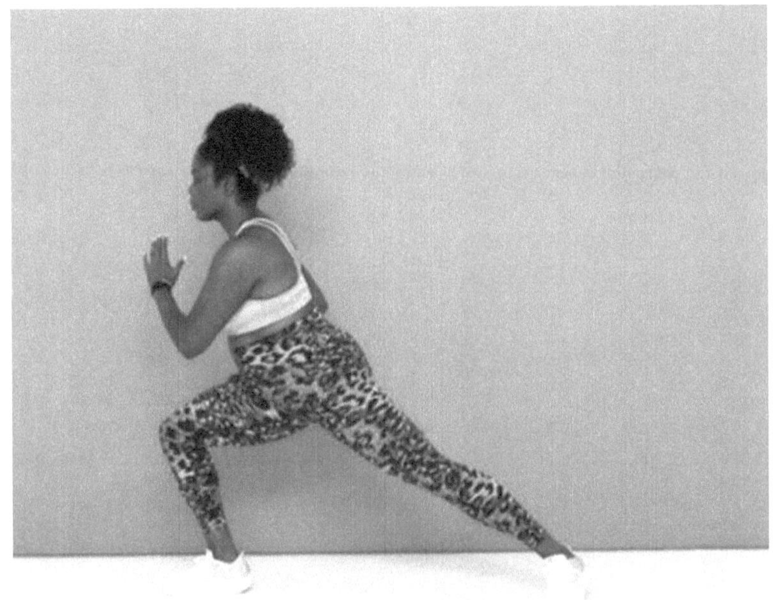

5

There Are No Burpees or Mountain Climbers in This Routine

Not a fan of burpees or mountain climbers? Then this HIIT workout is the routine for you. Created by Conlon, this total-body bodyweight workout gets you moving in multiple planes of motion to work all your different muscle groups. The exercises she chose—moves like the lateral shuffle and explosive crab reach—allow you to move at a pace where you can really ramp up the intensity, which is vital for HIIT workouts. Hint: Try performing each move 10 times on its own at a comfortable intensity before moving into the workout, so you are familiar with any new exercises.Try the workout.

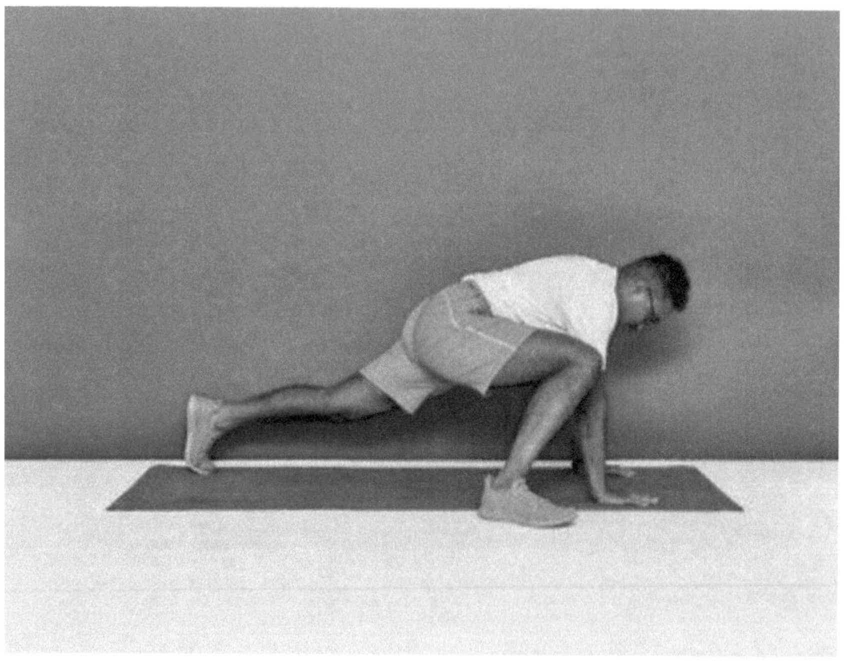

6

A 4-Move 30-Minute Cardio Workout

With this full-body at-home cardio workout, which was created by Eisinger, the goal is to move through three moves—froggers, bird-dog crunches, and a three-point toe touch—as quickly as possible. This 30-minute workout doubles as a cardio routine (no running required), so give it a shot if you are looking to get sweaty. You can choose rest-work periods based off your fitness level, so it's a great workout for those who are just getting started.

Try the workout.

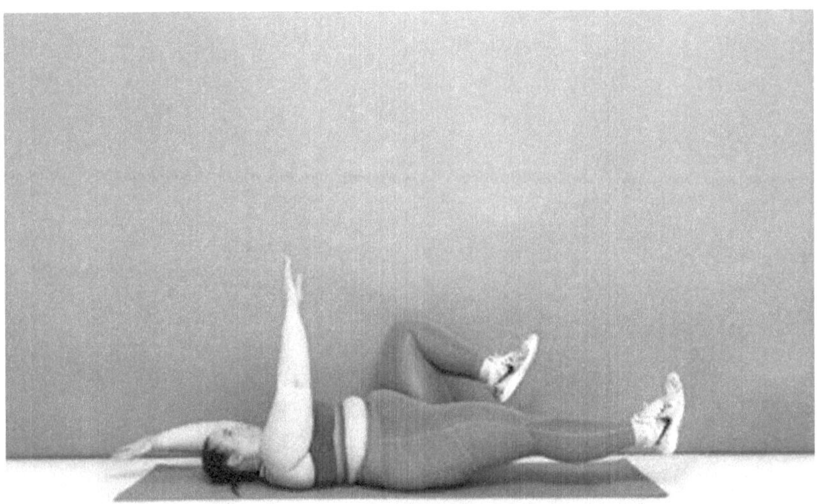

7

An Abs Workout That's Done in 8 Minutes

The good thing about abs workouts is that they're pretty easy to do at home without any equipment. The not-so-good part? Abs workouts can be superhard, which is why we're all for one that's over in eight minutes. With this at-home workout, which was created by Amy Marturana Winderl, C.P.T., you'll spend 30 seconds on five separate exercises, including dead bug, forearm plank rock, and plank up-down, taking no rest between the moves until the circuit is complete. After three rounds, your abs will definitely be burning.

Try the workout.

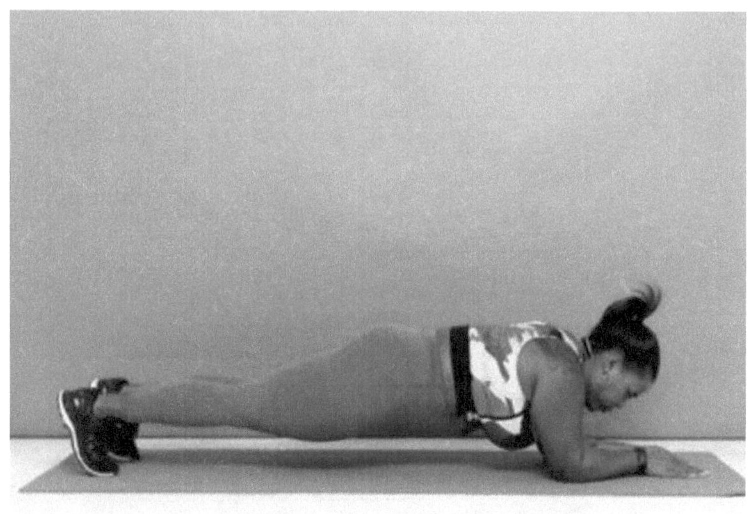

8

A 5-Minute Plank Workout That Challenges More Than Your Core

Planks are known for working your abs, but if you do them right, you'll seriously challenge your shoulders, legs, and butt too. Created by Marturana Winderl, this bodyweight workout uses five variations of the plank, including plank up-downs (which light up your shoulders and triceps) and plank jacks (to give a cardio element). Check out these tips to make a plank more effective before you get started, so you can make sure you are making the most of every exercise. Try the workout.

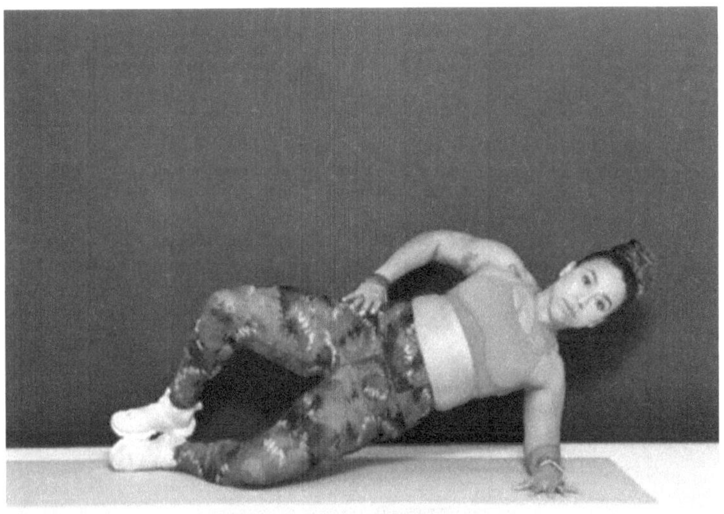

9

The 4-Move Bodyweight Workout That'll Seriously Work Your Butt

Sure, there are some kinds of equipment that work really well for butt exercises—we're looking at you, mini-bands—but you actually don't *need* anything at all (besides your bodyweight) to get your glutes working. This four-move workout, which was created by Cori Lefkowith, NASM-certified personal trainer and owner of Redefining Strength in Costa Mesa, California, proves you don't need any equipment for a good butt workout. Moves like frog bridges and straight-leg fire hydrant ensure you are working your gluteus maximus, medius, and minimus. Try the workout.

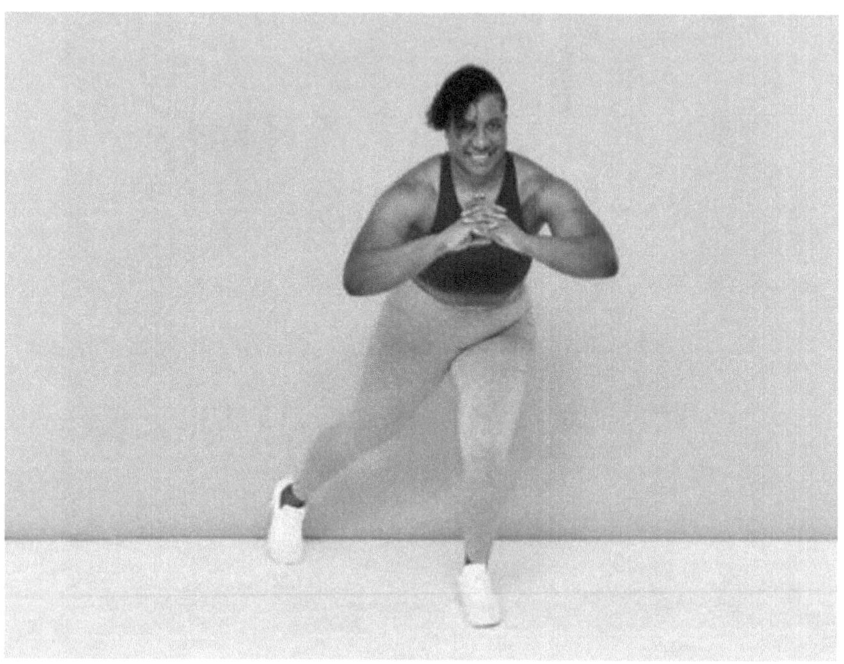

10

A 3-Move Cardio Workout for Beginners

There are only three simple moves in this workout created by Eisinger—the skater, three-point toe touch, and flutter kick—but it's a great way for you to get the moves down and ease into at-home workouts. If you're just getting started, try each move for 30 seconds with 30 seconds of rest. As you get more comfortable with exercising, you can increase your work time and decrease your rest for more of a cardio challenge.

Try the workout.

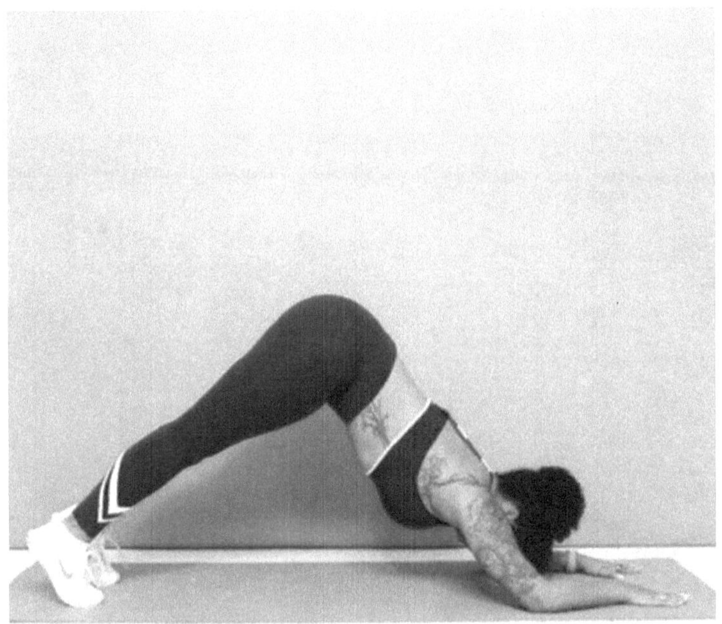

11

A Core Workout That's Great for Your Arms

This workout, created by TruFusion trainer Alyssa West, primarily works your core, but thanks to exercises like the push-up, plank-to-dolphin, and diamond push-up, your arms will get a serious workout too. There are nine exercises in the workout, which seems like a lot, but it only takes 15 minutes to finish. Your shoulders and triceps will totally be feeling it by the time you're done.

Try the workout.

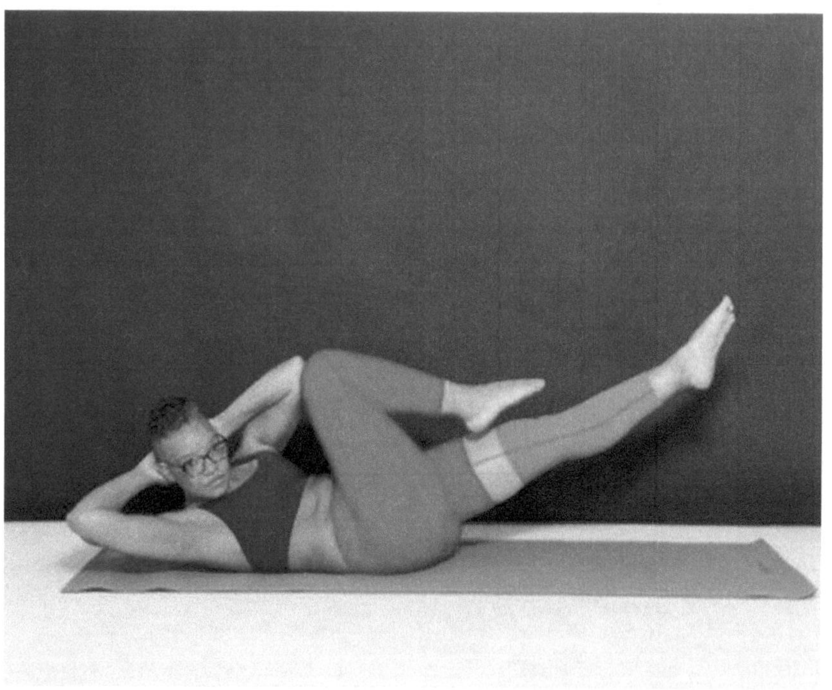

12

A 10-Minute Pilates Workout for Your Butt and Core

To really home in on specific muscles, sometimes small, controlled movements are key. That's one of the biggest benefits of Pilates-based workouts, and this routine, which was created by Manuela Sanchez, certified Pilates instructor at Club Pilates in Brooklyn, uses that to its full advantage. You can do this circuit once or twice as its own workout, but it's also great to really get your glutes muscles warmed up for a more leg-intensive workout. Try the workout.

Back and Biceps Workout for Strength and Muscle

This back and biceps workout focuses on building strength and lean muscle tissue in the lats, lower back, rhomboids, both heads of the biceps, shoulders, and the forearms. The workout is geared for those who have some experience using gym equipment and practicing good form.

The workout includes supersets, which means you'll do two exercises for the same muscle group back-to-back, then rest and repeat one or more times, using enough weight that you can only complete 10 to 12 repetitions per set. Supersets are great for those who are short on time but want to do several different exercises.

Safety and Precautions

Check with your healthcare provider if you have any current injuries, illnesses, or other conditions. You should also seek medical guidance if you are returning to exercise after pregnancy or injury or if you are prone to back pain.

Overview

Total Time: 30–45 minutes

Level: Intermediate to advanced

Equipment Needed: Dumbbells; a barbell with weight plates; a chair, weight bench, or ball; and a resistance band

What to Expect: You'll be performing four supersets total. Two supersets focus on the back muscles but also help to strengthen the arms and shoulders. Then you'll do two supersets that focus on the biceps.

For each exercise, choose a weight that allows you to finish each set with good form. The last rep should be very difficult, but not impossible. Perform the exercises in each set, rest for 30 to 60 seconds, and repeat.

For a lighter workout, complete each superset one time. For a more challenging workout, repeat each superset for a total of three times. You can vary the length of the workout by changing the number of sets that you complete.

Warm Up

Begin with a 5-minute warm-up of light cardio. If you have access to a treadmill, walk or jog at an easy to moderate intensity. You can also use a stationary bike or simply walk in place.

After completing your short cardio segment, complete a series of back extensions to further prepare the muscles in your back.

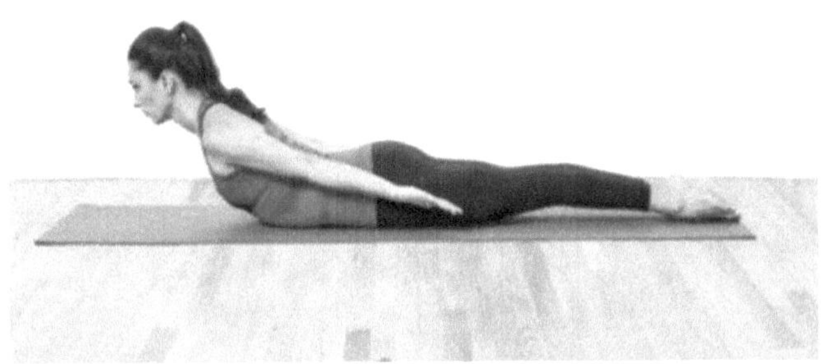

Ben Goldstein

Back Extensions

A back extension can be performed on a <u>machine at your local health club</u>. To perform the back extension at home without equipment, follow these steps.

Lie face down with hands alongside your body with palms facing up.

Lift upper body off the ground a few inches, keeping head and neck in alignment.

Hold for two counts.

Lower and repeat 10–15 times

Superset #1

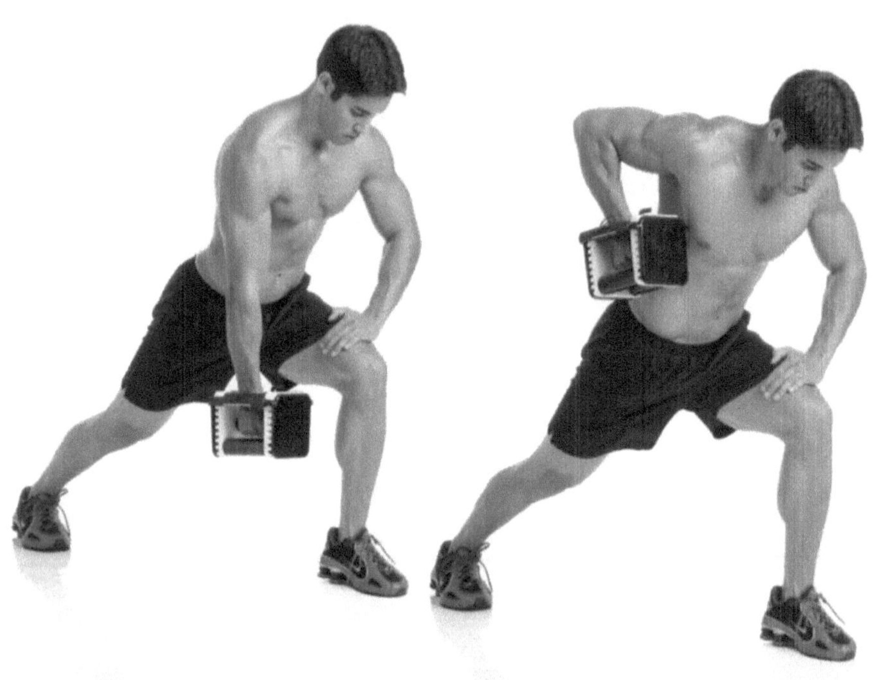

For your first superset, you'll perform two variations of a row exercise to work the large muscles in the back. Your shoulders and arms will also benefit from these movements.

One-Armed Row

You'll need heavy dumbbells for this exercise.

Place your left foot a few feet in front of you with your knee bent, and hold a heavy weight in your right hand. The palm should be facing the midline of the body.

Keeping the back strong and the core tight, engage the muscles in your back to pull the elbow up in a rowing motion until it is level with your torso.

Lower and repeat for 10–12 reps, then switch sides.

<u>Build Your Back With a One-Arm Row</u>

Barbell High Row

Begin this exercise standing tall (feet hip-width apart) with a barbell on the floor in front of you. If you are adding weight to the bar, be sure that the plates are secured with a collar. If you don't have a barbell, simply hold one dumbbell in each hand. When you are ready to begin, pick up the barbell with an overhand grip, palms facing your thighs.

Bend your knees slightly and hinge at the hips, bringing the torso forward until your back is almost parallel to the floor. Let the barbell hang in front of you.

Squeeze your shoulder blades together and engage the middle and upper back as you pull the weight toward your chest.

Lower the barbell and repeat for 10–12 reps.

After completing the barbell high row, repeat superset #1.

Superset #2

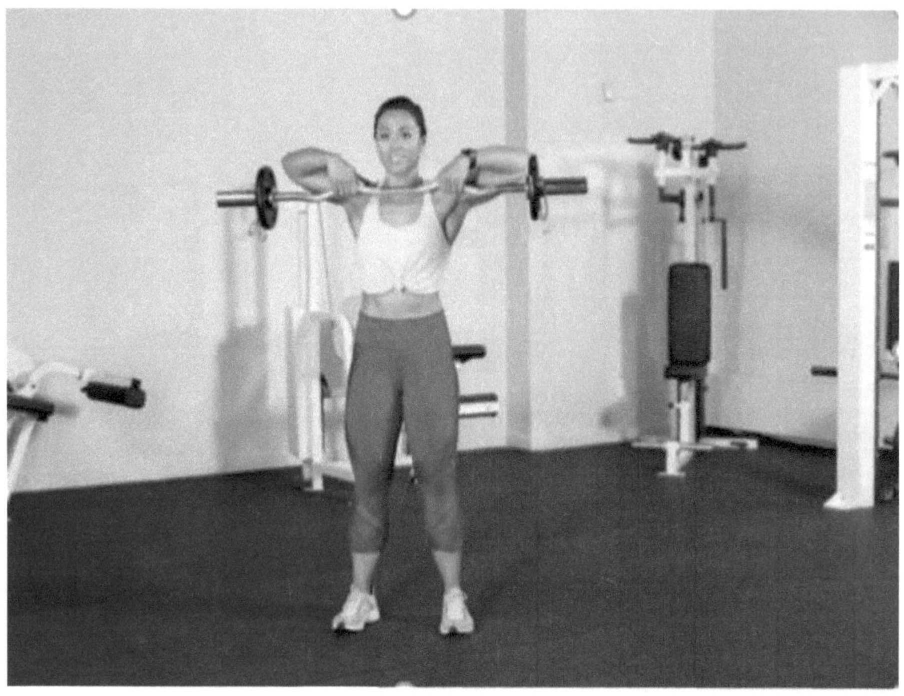

For your second superset, you'll perform two more row variations to continue to work the back and the shoulders.

Upright Row

This exercise is usually performed with a barbell, but you can use dumbbells (one in each hand) if a barbell is not available. Start by standing tall, holding the barbell with an overhand grip so that your palms face your body. Hands should be shoulder-width apart.

Keeping the abdominals engaged, lift the barbell straight up toward your chin, leading with the elbows and keeping the bar close to the body.

Pause when the bar reaches shoulder height.

Return the barbell back to the starting position and repeat 10–12 times.

<u>How to Work Your Back With the Upright Row</u>

Alternating T-Pulls and Y-Pulls

You'll use a resistance band for this exercise. If you are working out in a gym or at home and have access to <u>TRX straps</u>, you can do this exercise standing and using the straps instead.

If you are using bands, start seated with your legs extended in front of you. Loop the band around both feet, holding one end of the band in each hand. Make sure there is very little slack in the band.

Keeping a strong, tall back, engage your middle and upper back and open your arms out to a T-shape.

Return to the starting position and repeat, but this time, bring your arms up and out into a Y-shape.

Return to the starting position and continue alternating T-pulls and Y-pulls for 10–12 repetitions.

After completing the alternating T-pulls and Y-pulls, repeat superset #2.

Superset #3

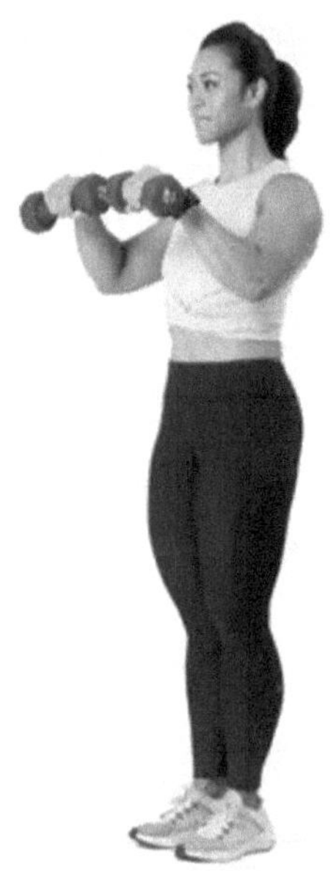

Your supersets will now begin to focus on the front of the body, specifically the biceps. You'll begin with these two standing exercises that are variations of the basic biceps curl.

Barbell Curl

Start with your feet hip-width apart and abdominals engaged. Hold the barbell in front of you with an underhand grip, palms facing forward. If you don't have a barbell, simply grab two dumbbells and hold one in each hand.

Keeping your upper arms stable and shoulders relaxed, bend at the elbow and lift the barbell so that it approaches your shoulders. The elbows should stay tucked in close to the ribs.

Lower the barbell to the starting position and repeat 10–12 times.

Reverse Curl

To perform a reverse dumbbell curl, you'll hold one dumbbell in each hand using an overhand grip. Your palms should be facing your thighs when you begin.

Bending at the elbow, lift the weights up toward your shoulders but pause when your elbows reach a 90-degree bend (or slightly higher).

Slowly lower the weights with control to the starting position.

Repeat the exercise for 10–12 repetitions.

How to Do a Reverse Bicep Curl

After completing your reverse curls, repeat superset #3.

Superset #4

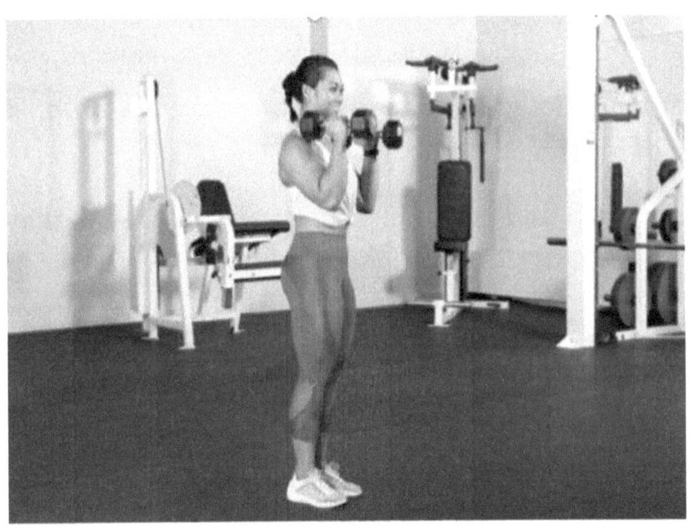

This last superset provides two more exercises to work the biceps. You'll need dumbbells to perform each exercise.

Hammer Curls

Start standing with feet about hip-width apart, holding one dumbbell in each hand with your palms facing your thighs.

Keeping your upper arms in a fixed position, bend at the elbow and lift your lower arms up and toward your shoulders.

At the top of the movement, your thumbs will be close to your shoulders, palms facing in toward the midline of the body.

Lower the weights to the starting position and repeat 10–12 times.

<u>Perfect Dumbbell Pullover Technique and Tips</u>

Concentration Curl

This exercise allows you to focus on one arm at a time. You'll start seated on a chair or weight bench. Place a dumbbell in your right hand with your elbow extended straight down but propped against the inside of your right thigh.

Engage the bicep and curl the weight towards your shoulder. Keep the elbow pressed against the right leg so it remains stable.

Lower the weight to the starting position and repeat 10–12 times. Repeat with the left arm.

Home Dumbbell Workout Plan

How To Warm Up

One of the advantages of home workouts is that you don't have to spend any time travelling to and from the gym, which means you definitely have the time to get a thorough warm-up in before you tackle one of the sessions below.

You only need to spend a few minutes warming up before the workout to be firing on all cylinders from the off, rather than creaking your way through the first couple of sets with cold muscles. Warming up also reduces your risk of injury during a workout, and it should help reduce any muscle soreness you experience in the days afterwards.

The key to a good warm-up is to work the muscles you're intending to use in the workout itself. There's little point in jogging on the spot or doing jumping jacks if you're about to do a weights session. Instead try this routine, which involves seven stretches that target muscles all over the body, followed by movements that mirror the workout you're about to perform. Your best bet is simply to perform the exercises you intend to do in your workout using light weights or no weight at all, which will get your muscles used to the relevant movements before you challenge them with added resistance.

Workout 1: Monday

1 Dumbbell swing

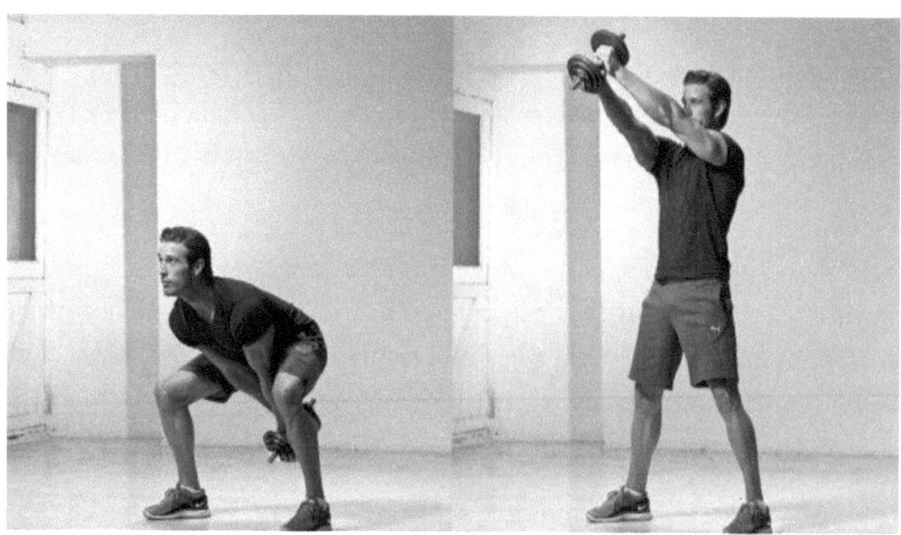

Sets 3 **Reps** 10 **Rest** 60sec

Send the dumbbell between your legs by hingeing at the hips, then push your glutes forwards powerfully so you use hip drive to raise the dumbbell to shoulder height. Reverse the movement to the start and go straight into the next rep.

2 Overhead squat

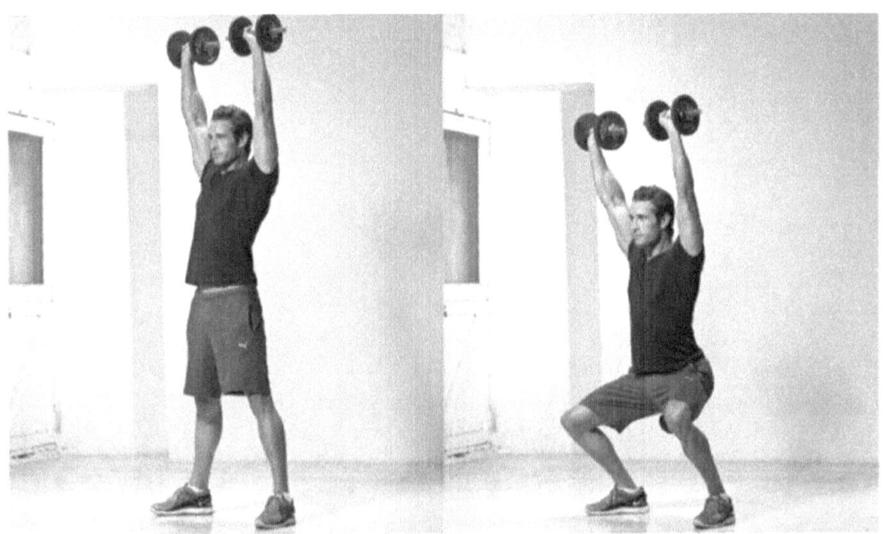

Sets 3 **Reps** 10 **Rest** 60sec

Start with both weights held directly overhead, then simultaneously bend at the hips and knees to lower into a squat, without letting the weights come forwards.

3 Side lunge

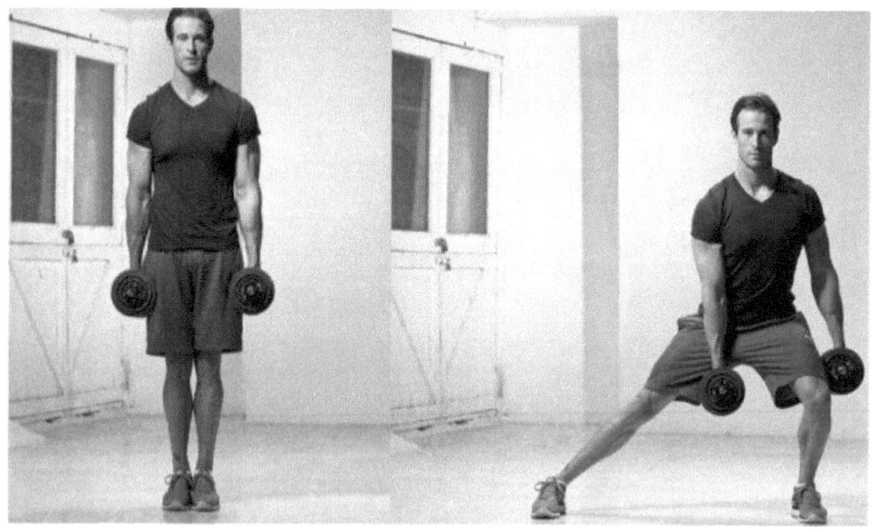

Sets 3 **Reps** 8 each side **Rest** 60sec

Start with a dumbbell in each hand, then take a big step to one side and bend your leading knee, keeping your foot pointing forwards and your knee in line with your toes. Push off your leading foot to return to the start, then take a big step the other way to repeat the move. Alternate sides with each rep.

4 Press-up renegade row

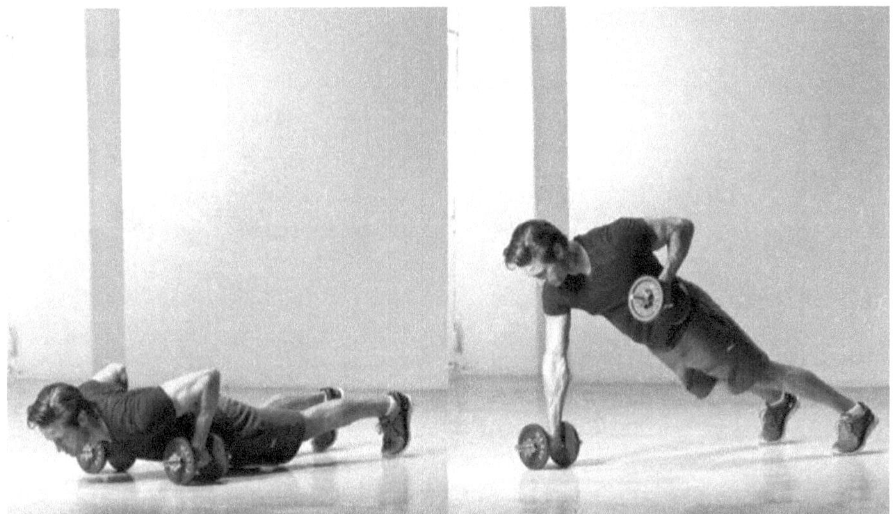

Sets 3 **Reps** 8 **Rest** 60sec

Holding a dumbbell in each hand, perform a press-up then at the top, row one dumbbell up to your side. Lower the weight, then row the other dumbbell up to complete one rep.

5 Leg raise

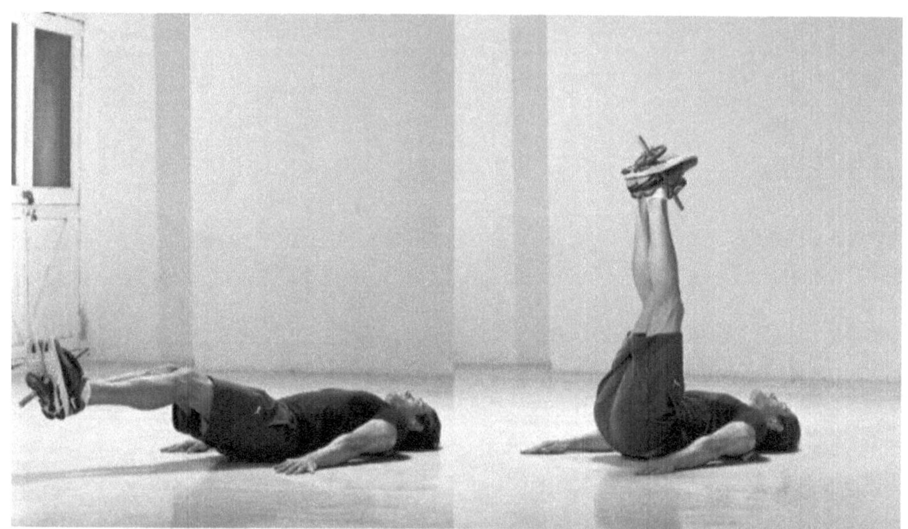

Sets 3 **Reps** 10 **Rest** 60sec

Hold a dumbbell between your feet with your heels raised slightly off the ground. Keeping your legs straight, raise them until they are vertical, then lower slowly under control without letting your heels touch the floor.

Workout 2: Wednesday

Like the first workout of the week, this session focuses on functional movements. And you can't get more functional than a power snatch, which involves shifting a weight from a low position to above your head in one explosive move. The next move is the jump squat, which is a safe way of improving power just as you start to fatigue in the workout. The two abs moves at the end of the session are among the most effective exercises you can do in your quest to develop a rock-hard six-pack.

1 Power snatch

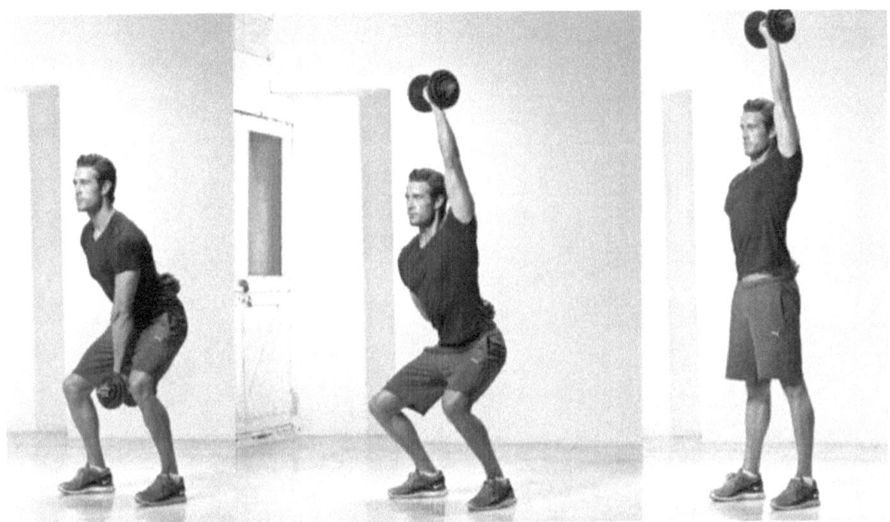

Sets 3 **Reps** 10 **Rest** 60sec

Hold a dumbbell in one hand between your legs with your knees bent. Explosively extend your hips, knees and ankles to raise the weight overhead. Once your body is straight from head to toe, drop into a half squat to "catch" the weight overhead, then stand up straight.

2 Squat press (or thruster)

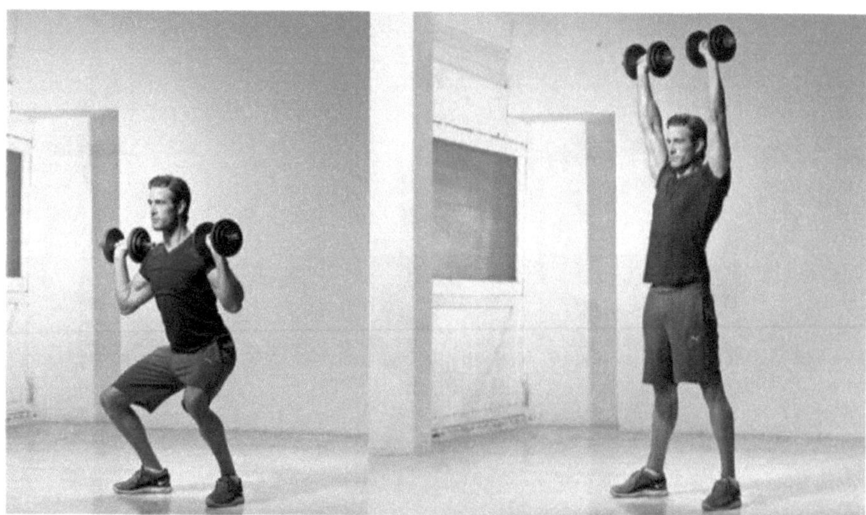

Sets 3 **Reps** 10 **Rest** 60sec

Start with the dumbbells at shoulder level and lower into a squat, then stand up and press the weights directly overhead. Lower the weights and return to the start position.

3 Jump squat

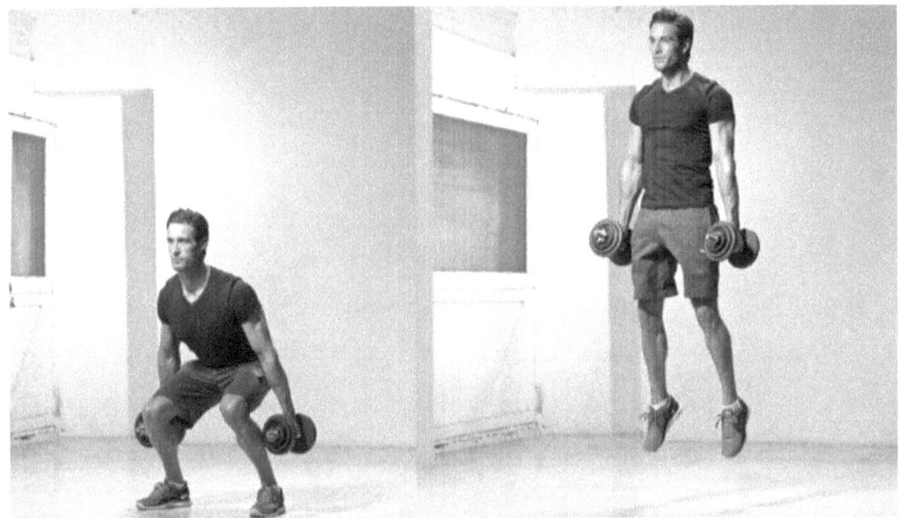

Sets 3 **Reps** 6 **Rest** 60sec

Start with the dumbbells by your sides and lower into a half squat. Jump straight up off the ground, land softly and go straight into the next rep.

4 Windmill

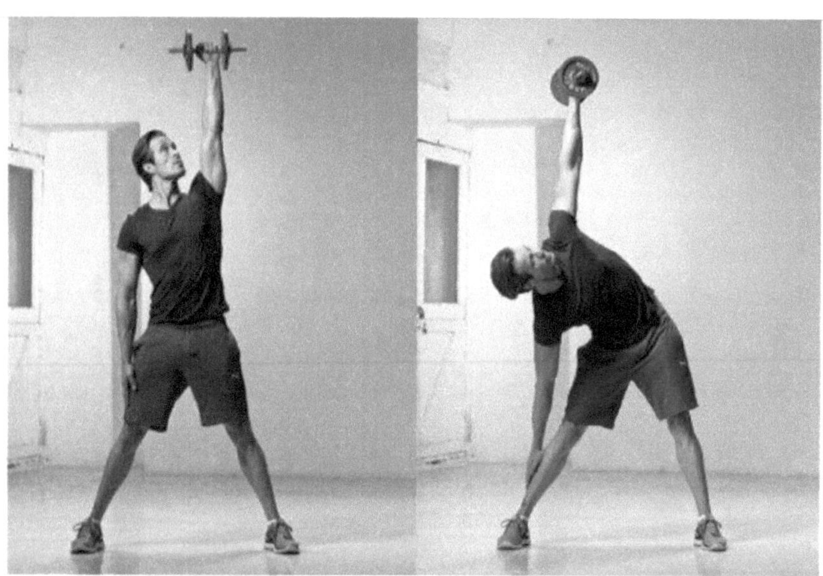

Sets 2 **Reps** 10 each side **Rest** 60sec

Hold a dumbbell overhead, then bend at the waist by guiding one hand down your leg. Make sure you keep looking at the weight throughout the move.

5 Roll-out

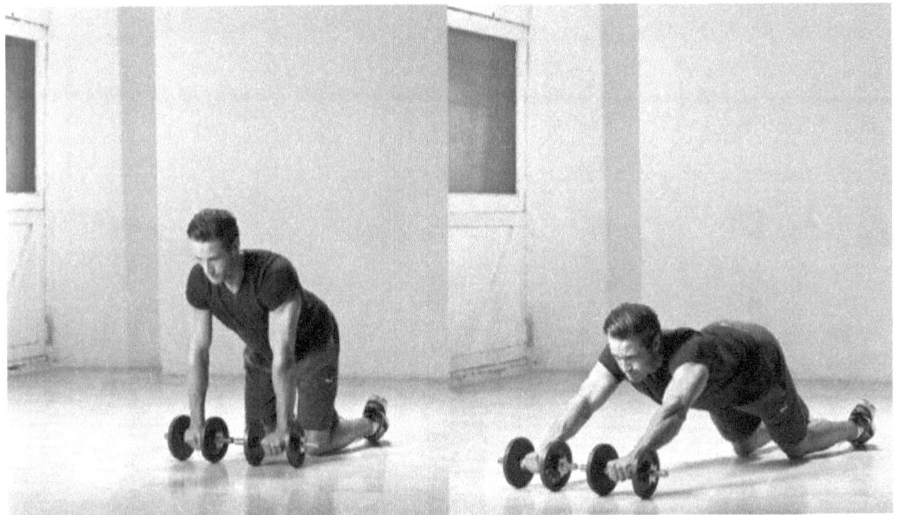

Sets 3 **Reps** 10 **Rest** 60sec

Kneel with the dumbbells below your shoulders. Roll the weights forwards as far as you can, using your abs to control the movement, then return to the start.

Workout 3: Friday

It's the final workout of the week – but the moves don't get any easier. In fact, the first one may be the most challenging you've ever attempted. It may not look particularly complex or heavy, but pressing weights directly overhead from a squat position requires impressive levels of mobility and control. The session ends with Turkish get-ups, where you go from lying down to standing up with the weight overhead. It's so good that it's almost an entire workout in itself.

1 Back of steel

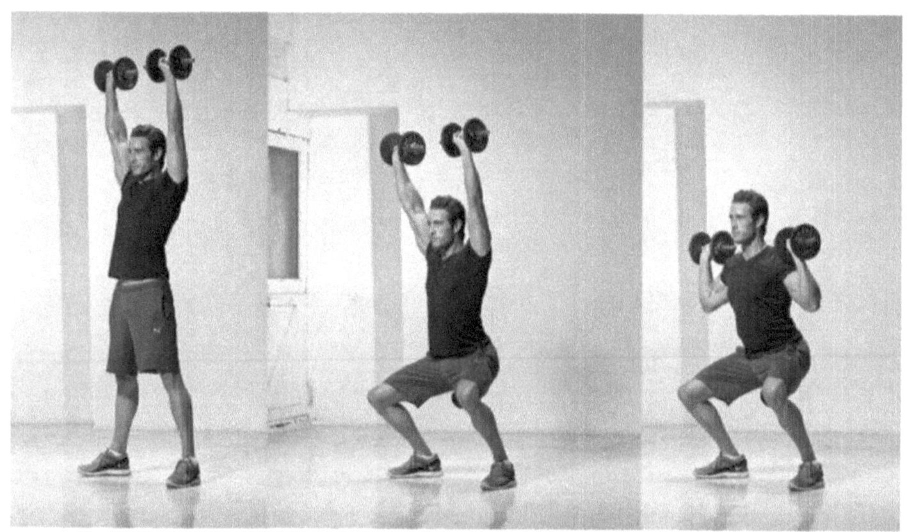

Sets 3 **Reps** 10 **Rest** 60sec

Start with the dumbbells above your head, then lower into an overhead squat. While still in a squat position, lower the weights to shoulder height, then press them overhead. Continue to repeat the lowering and pressing movement while in a squat.

2 One-leg Romanian deadlift

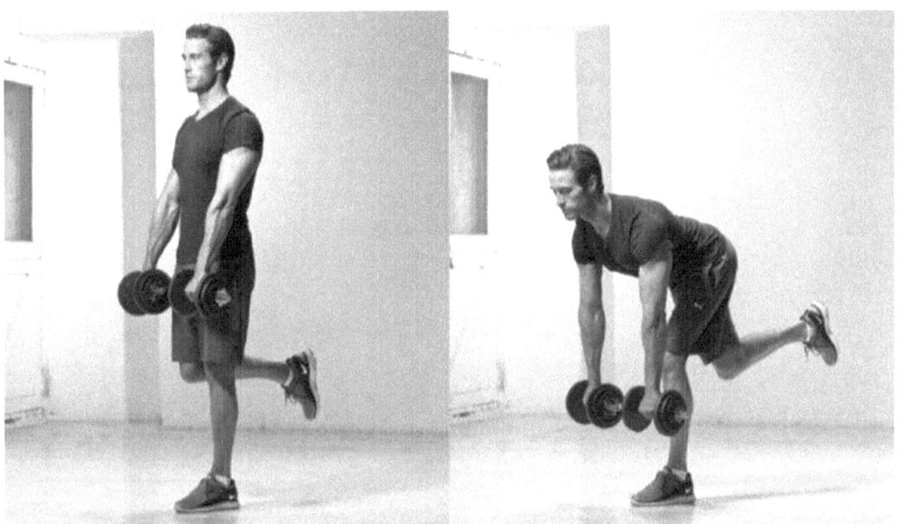

Sets 2 **Reps** 10 each side **Rest** 60sec

Stand on one leg with the weights hanging down by your thighs. Hinge at the hips to lower the weights towards the floor, keeping them close to your leg – don't come too far forwards because that will put strain on your lower back.

3 One-leg squat

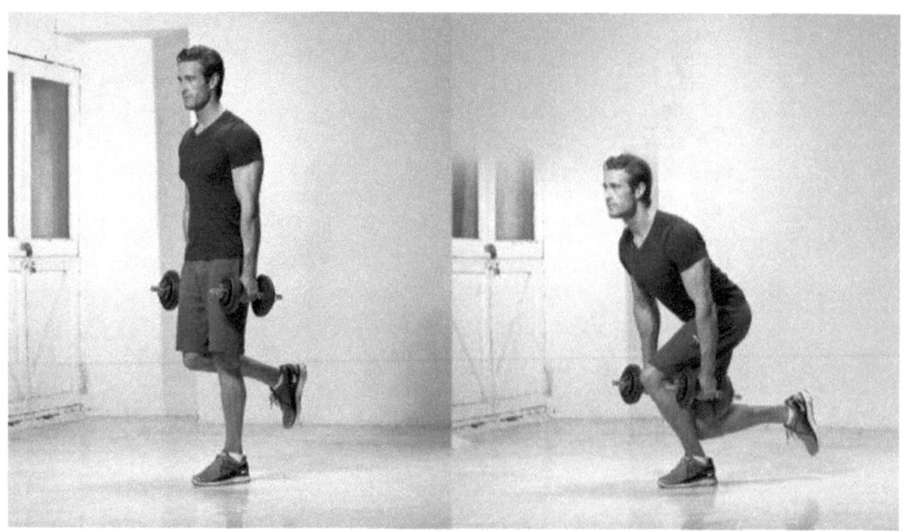

Sets 2 **Reps** 6-8 each side **Rest** 60sec

Stand on one leg with the dumbbells by your sides. Keeping your chest up, bend at the hips and knees to lower into a single-leg squat. Press back up to the start. Complete all the reps on that leg, then switch to the other leg.

4 Woodchop lunge

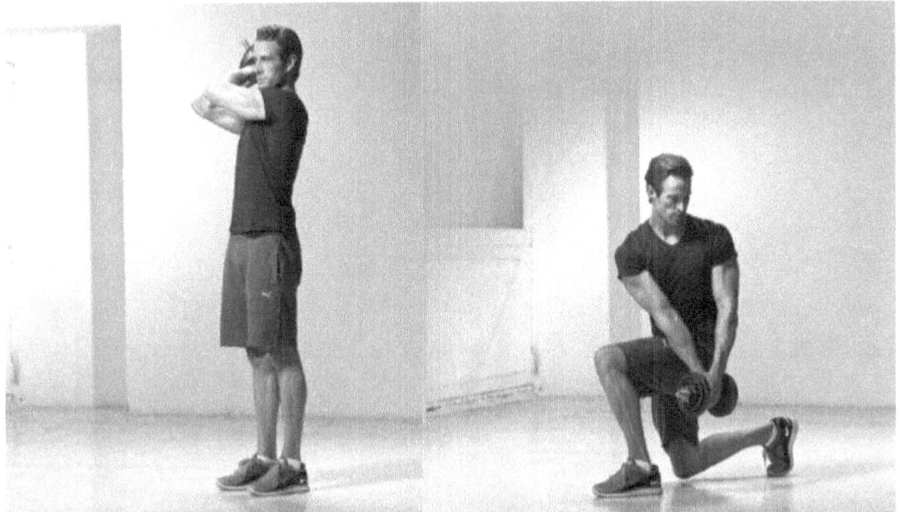

Sets 3 **Reps** 8 each side **Rest** 60sec

Start with a dumbbell over one shoulder. Lunge forwards with the opposite leg and simultaneously bring the weight down and across your body. Do all the reps on one side, then swap sides.

5 Turkish get-up

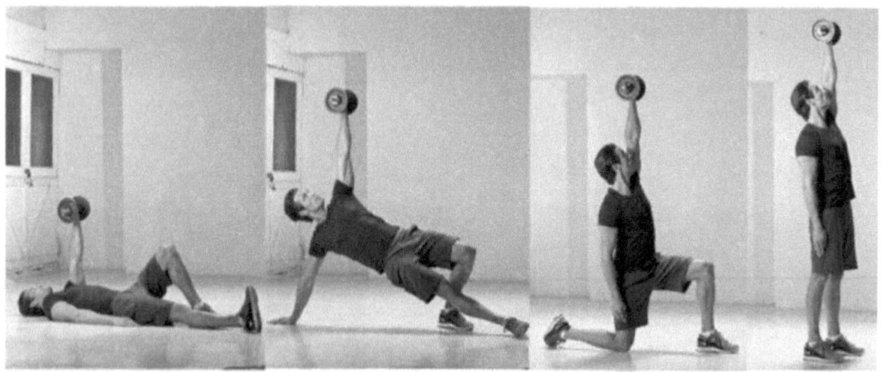

Sets 2 **Reps** 6 each side **Rest** 60sec

Lie on the floor holding a weight above your face. Bend your knee on that side then come up onto your elbow, then your hand and push your hips off the floor. Bring your straight leg back below your body, then take your hand off the floor and stand up.

Workouts to Build Muscle

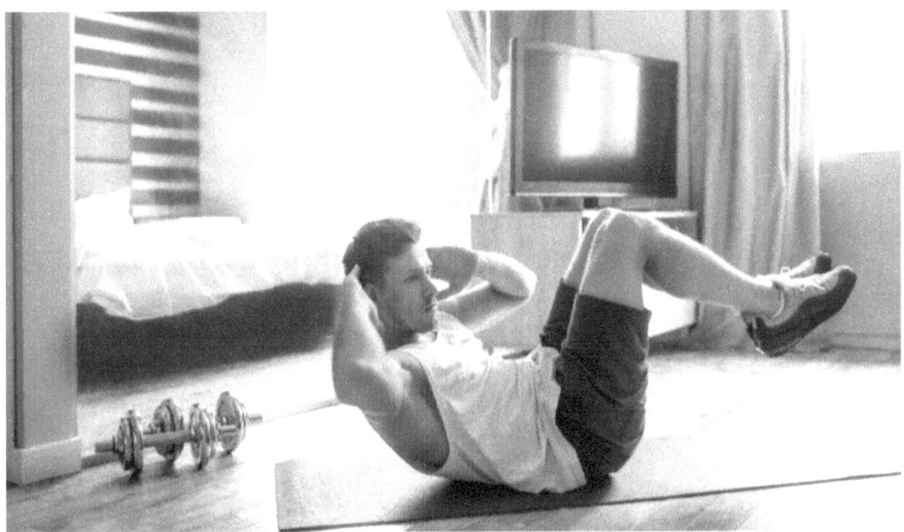

You put in long hours at work, or maybe even work overnight shifts. You're tight on money. You want to spend downtime with friends. A hurricane or global pandemic has you barricaded in your home. Whatever the reason, there are times when you just can't make it to the gym. We've all been there. And so long as you don't use that as an excuse to skip workouts, you're golden. There are plenty of at-home workouts to build muscle.

There's no reason you can't build mass, strength, and size at home. It won't take all day either. Training with minimal equipment, or even just bodyweight, is enough to get you in the shape you want.

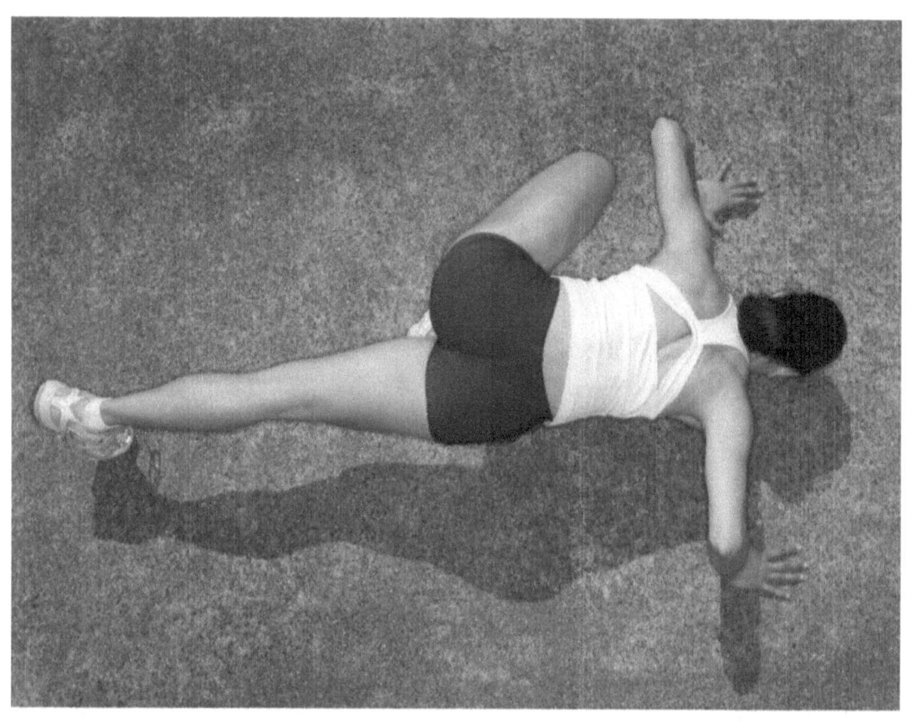

1. Bodyweight Spiderman

Directions: Perform all A exercises, then all B exercises, then all C exercises.

A1)	Feet-elevated	Pike	Pushup
Sets:			4
Reps:			12
Rest:		60	seconds

Get into a pike position—arms straight and legs straight with your hips high in the air—with your feet on a sturdy elevated surface, like a box. Slowly lower yourself, and drive back up.

A2)	Alternating	Split	Squat	Jump

Sets: 4
Reps: 10   (each   leg)
Rest: 60   seconds

Start in a split stance. Squat down and explode into the air, switch legs, and land in the opposite stance. Alternate quickly, and jump as high as you can each time.

B1)   Spiderman   Crawl
Sets: 6
Reps: 10
Rest: 30   seconds

Start in a pushup position. Crawl forward by taking a large step with your right arm and left leg at the same time—get low to the ground and swing your left knee so that it almost touches your right elbow. Alternate sides and keep your body low to the ground. To increase the difficulty, crawl backwards.

B2)   Spiderman   Pushups
Sets: 6
Reps   (each   leg)
Rest: 30   seconds

Start in a pushup position. As you lower yourself, pull one knee toward that same-side's elbow. As you rise, bring your leg back. Repeat on the other side and continue alternating.

B3)   Single-Leg   Box   Squats
Sets: 6
Reps: 6
Rest: 60   sec.

Start by facing away from a bench or box. Lift one leg, sit

back onto the bench, and come up without putting your other leg down. To make it harder, lower the bench.

C1)   Alternating   Side-plank
Sets: 4
Reps: 5   (each   side)
Rest: 30   seconds
Lie on your side, and place your forearm on the ground, perpendicular to your body. Keep your body straight, your glutes squeezed, and your shoulders pulled back. Don't let your hips sag. Twist your body toward the ground, switch arms, and do a side-plank facing the other way.

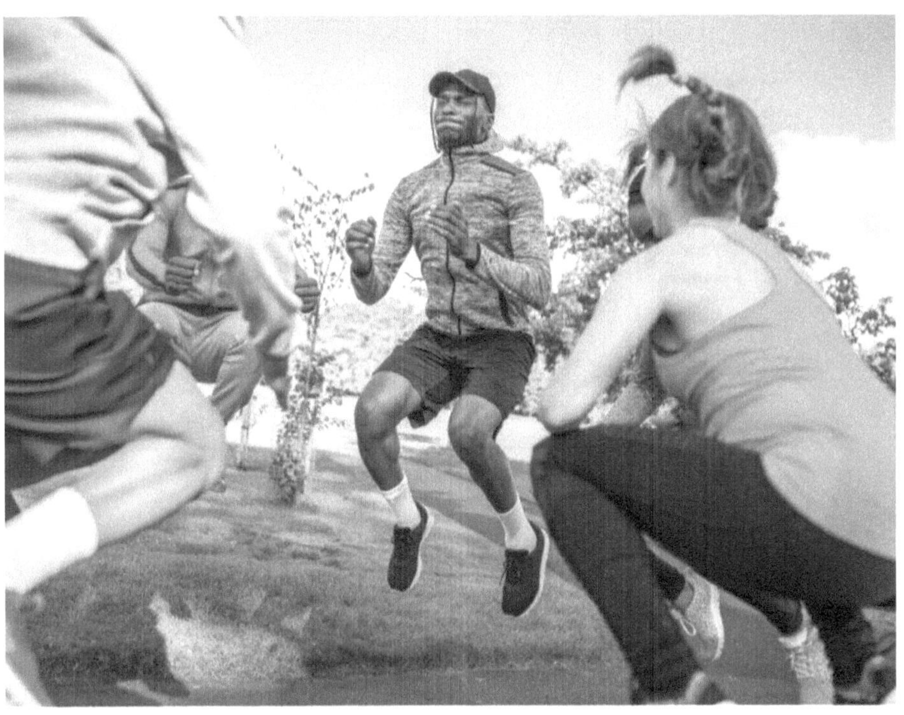

2. Bodyweight Squats

Directions:

Do all A exercises then all B exercises. For example, you'll do A1 (siff squat) then A2 (prisoner hold jump squats and then start over with the siff squat for the second set. Do the same for the B and C exercises.

The workout

A1.	Siff	Squat
Sets:		6
Reps:		15
No		rest

Stand shoulder-width apart with your feet slightly turned out. Get onto the balls of your feet, and stay there throughout. Squat down, sitting back and spreading your knees apart. Once you descend below parallel, drive back up.

A2.	Prisoner	Hold	Jump	Squats
Sets:				6
Reps:				15
Rest:		60		sec.

Stand shoulder-width apart with your feet slightly turned out. Places your hands behind your head. Squat down, sitting back and spreading your knees apart. Keep your weight on your heels. Once you descend below parallel, explode up and jump as high as you can.

B1.	Feet-elevated	Pike	Pushups
Sets:			4
Reps:			8
Rest:		60	sec.

Get into a pike position—arms straight and legs straight with your hips high in the air—with your feet on a bench or small box. Slowly lower yourself, and drive back up.

B2.	Alternating	Split	Squat	Jumps
Sets:				4
Reps:		5		each
Rest:		60		sec.

Start in a split stance. Squat down and explode into the air, switching legs, and landing in the opposite stance. Alternate quickly, and jump as high as you can each time.

C1.	Salute	Planks

Sets: 3
Reps: 5   (each   arm)
Rest: 30   sec.
Get into a plank position. Bring one hand to your forehead in a salute position, and hold for three seconds before switching arms. Prevent your hips from twisting as you salute.

C2.   Body   Saw
Sets: 3
Reps: 10
Rest: 30   sec.
Get into a plank position with only your feet on Valslides. Squeeze your glutes, and tighten your core. Then, push your body backward with your forearms as far as you can. Pull yourself back to the starting position, and repeat. The farther back you push, the harder you hit your core.

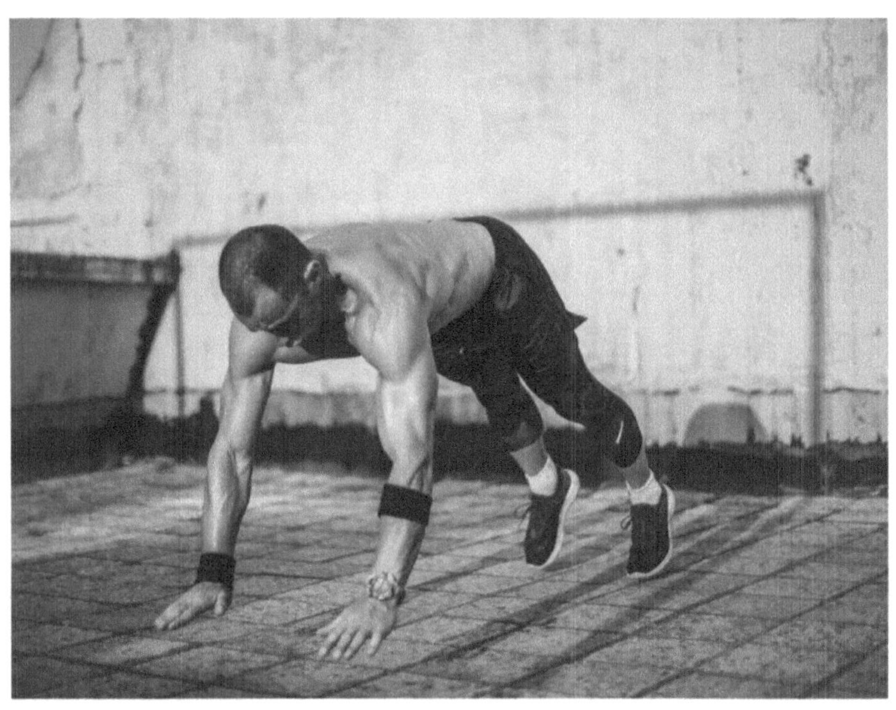

3. Burpee Finisher

Directions: Perform all A exercises, then all B exercises, then all C exercises.

A1.   L-pullups
Sets: 5
Reps: 8
Rest: 60   seconds
Grab a pullup bar, and lift your legs in front of you so your body forms an L. Hold this position and perform your pullups.

A2.   Feet-elevated   Pushups
Sets: 5

Reps: 15
Rest: 60   seconds
Perform a regular pushup with your feet on a small box or bench.

B1.   Skater   Squat
Sets: 4
Reps: 10   reps
Rest: 60   seconds
Start from a stand, and bend one foot behind you. Then, squat down while trying to touch the knee of the bent leg onto the ground behind you. Let your torso lean, and reach your arms forward as you descend.

B2.   Single-Leg   Box   Squats
Sets: 4
Reps: 10
Rest: 60   seconds
Start by facing away from a bench or box. Lift one leg, sit back onto the bench, and come up without putting your other leg down. To make it harder, lower the bench.

B3.   Valslide   Lateral   Squat
Sets: 4
Reps: (10   each   leg)
Rest: 60   seconds
Place one foot on a Valslide. Squat, and push your sliding leg directly out to the side while squatting down on your stationary leg. On your stationary leg, focus on sitting backward with your weight on your heel, keeping your chest tall, and keeping a neutral arch in your lower back.

C1.		Burpees
Sets:		4
Reps:		10
Rest:	30	seconds

Start in a pushup position. Do one pushup and, as you rise, explosively pull your knees toward your chest and place your feet underneath your chest. Then, jump as high as you can. Once you land, put your hands on the ground and kick your legs behind to return to a pushup position. Repeat as fast as you can.

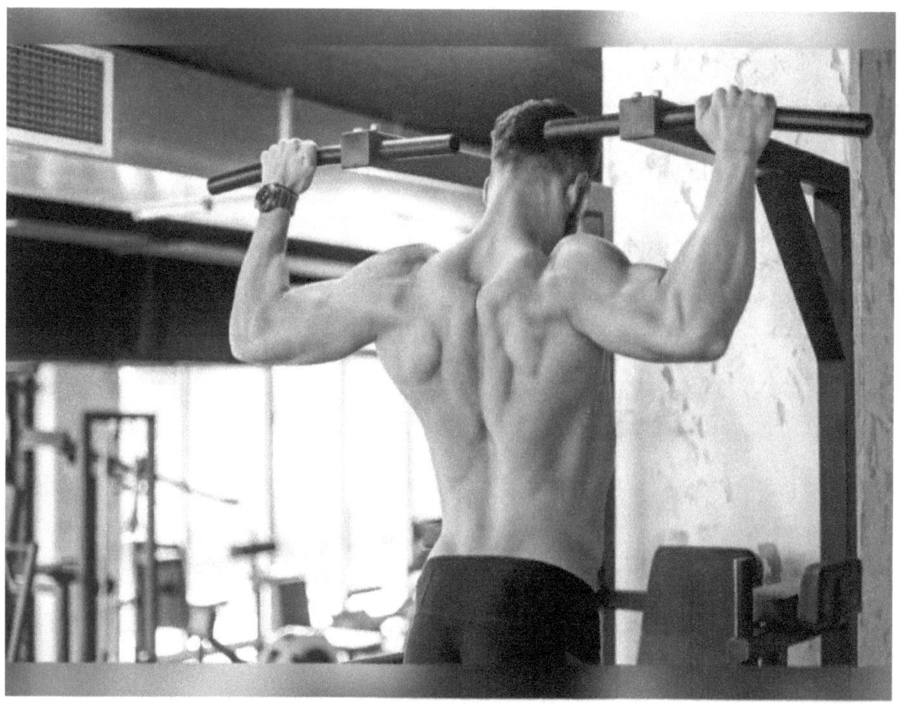

4. Pullup to Failure

Directions: Perform all A exercises, then all B exercises, then all C exercises.

A1. Wide-grip Pullups

Sets: 5

Reps: Until failure

Rest: 90 sec.

Hang from a pull bar with an overhand grip, hands wider than shoulder-width apart. Squeeze your shoulder blades together, and pull yourself up until your chin is over the bar.

B1. Single-leg Box Squats

Sets: 4

Reps: 12

Rest: 60 sec.

Start by facing away from a bench or box. Lift one leg, sit back onto the bench, and come up without putting your other leg down. To make it harder, lower the bench.

B2. Hip/thigh Extension

Sets: 4

Reps: 12

Rest: 60 sec.

Lie on your back and bend one knee so that it makes a 90° angle, and stick the other leg straight out. With your bent leg, squeeze your glute, push through your heel, push your hips up, and keep your hips level as you rise. Keep your straight leg extended throughout the exercise and keep it inline with your torso.

B3. Pushup + Overhead Reach

Sets: 4

Reps: 6 (each side)
Rest: 60 sec.
Place one palm on a slideboard or slider. From the pushup position, descend into a pushup while simultaneously reaching forward with the hand on the sliding surface. When you're at the bottom of the pushup, your sliding arm should be locked out.

C1. Forward Crawl
Sets: 5
Duration: 30 sec. crawling
Rest: 30 sec. — Start on all fours, with your shoulders directly above your hands, your hips above your knees, and your knees an inch above the ground. Crawl forward by taking a tiny step with your right arm and left leg at the same time, and then another step with your left arm and right leg. Alternate while keeping your hips low and your head up. To increase the difficulty, crawl backwards or laterally.

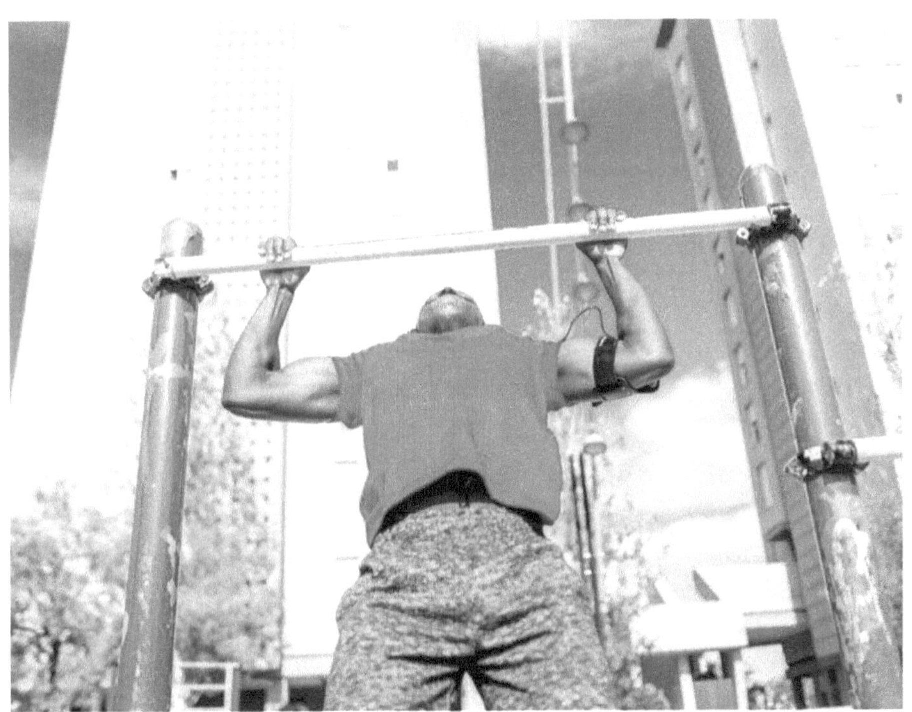

5. Chinup and Slider Workout

Directions: Perform all A exercises, then all B exercises, then all C exercises.

A1.	Slider	Leg	Curl
Sets:			6
Reps:			8
Rest:		60	sec.

Lie on your back with your feet on sliders. Start by squeezing your glutes and extending your hips. Then, curl your feet underneath your knees while keeping your hips extended and maintain a straight line from your shoulders to your knees. Remember: Every inch you curl your feet is another inch your hips need to rise.

B1.   Feet-elevated   Pushups
Sets: 5
Reps: 8
Rest: 60   sec.
Perform a regular pushup with your feet on a small box or bench.

B2.   Chinups
Sets: 5
Reps: 8
Rest: 60   sec.
Grab a pullup bar shoulder-width apart with a supinated grip. Squeeze your shoulder blades together, and pull your chest to the bar.

C1.   Alligator   Drags
Sets: 4
Reps: 10
Rest: 30   sec.
Place both feet on a slideboard or on separate Valslides. Get into pushup position with your glutes squeezed and core tight. While keeping your arms straight, march forward with your arms while dragging your legs behind you. Keep your legs straight.

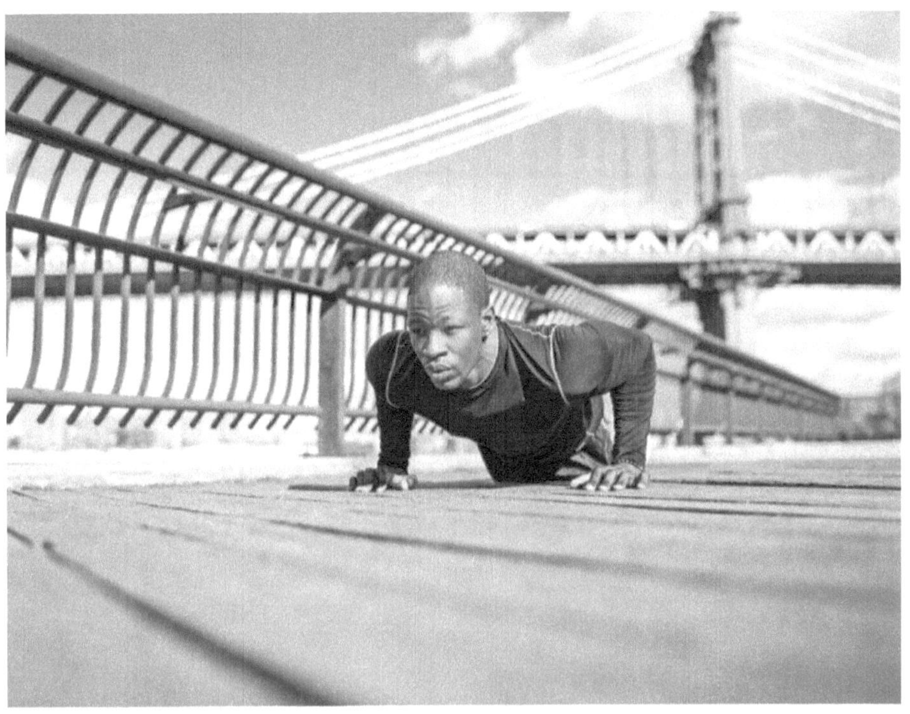

6. Full-body Bodyweight Workout (with warmup)

The warmup (will make total workout time greater than 20 minutes): Do all three exercises in a row, and then repeat the circuit again for a total of six sets.

1. Squat to Stand
Reps: 10

2. Alternating Lunges (with hands behind head)
Reps: 10 (each leg)

3. Lateral Lunges (hands in front)
Reps: 10 (each leg)

The workout: Do all A exercises, then all B exercises. For example, you'll do A1, then A2, then A3, and then start over with glute bridge marches for the second set. Do the same for the B exercises.

A1. Glute Bridge March
Sets: 2
Reps: 10 (each leg)

A2. Pushups
Sets: 2 Reps: As many as possible

A3. Bulgarian Split Squat (foot on chair, box, or bench)
Sets: 2 Reps: 12 (per leg)

B1. Donkey Kicks
Sets: 2 Reps: 12

B2. Plank to Pushup
Sets: 2 Reps: 12

B3. Straight Leg Situp (reach for ceiling)
Sets: 2 Reps: 10

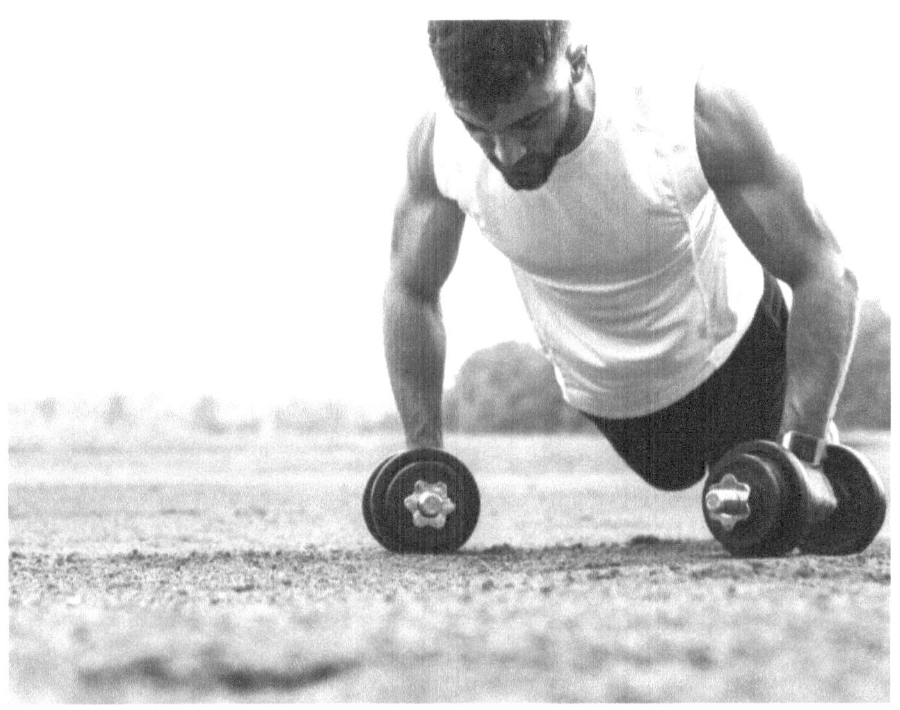

7. Dumbbell Workout

Directions: Do all A exercises then all B exercises. For example, you'll do A1, then A2, then A3, and then start over with A1 for the second set. Do the same for the B exercises.

A1.   Bulgarian   Split   Squat
Sets: 2
Reps: 6 (each leg)

A2.   Single   Arm   Dumbbell   Floor   Press
Sets: 2
Reps: 8   (each   arm)
Use a neutral grip and touch the dumbbell to your armpit on each

rep.

A3.   Chest-supported   Dumbbell   Row
Sets: 2
Reps: 10
Set bench to approximately 35° angle, stand with toes on floor and body facing bench. Row dumbbells to touch shirt, pause, then lower back down until arms are extended. If you don't have a bench, do standing bentover dumbbell rows.

B1.   Goblet   Squat
Sets: 2
Reps: 20

B2.   Dumbbell   Pushup
Sets: 2
Reps: AMRAP

B3.   Bentover   Reverse   Flye
Sets: 2
Reps: 12

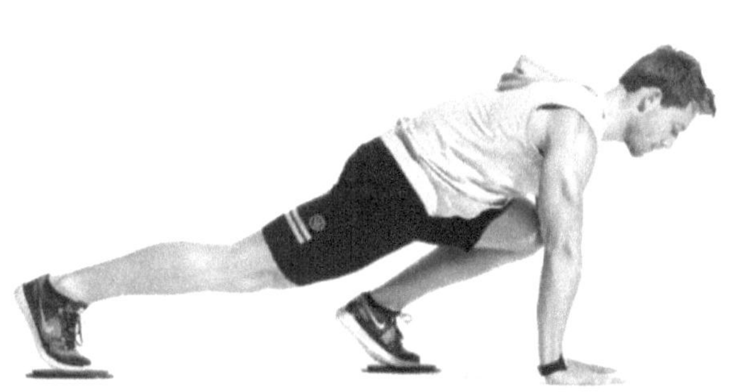

8. Valslide Workout

Directions: Do all A exercises then all B exercises. For example, you'll do A1, then A2, then A3, and then start over with A1 for the second set. Do the same for the B exercises.

A1.   Sliding   Reverse   Lunge
Sets: 2
Reps: 15

A2.   Bodysaw
Sets: 2
Reps: 15

A3.   Pushups
Sets: 2

Reps: 15

B1. Sliding Leg Curls
Sets: 2
Reps: 15

B2. Sliding Pike
Sets: 2
Reps: 15

B3. Sliding Mountain Climbers
Sets: 2
Reps: 15 (each leg)

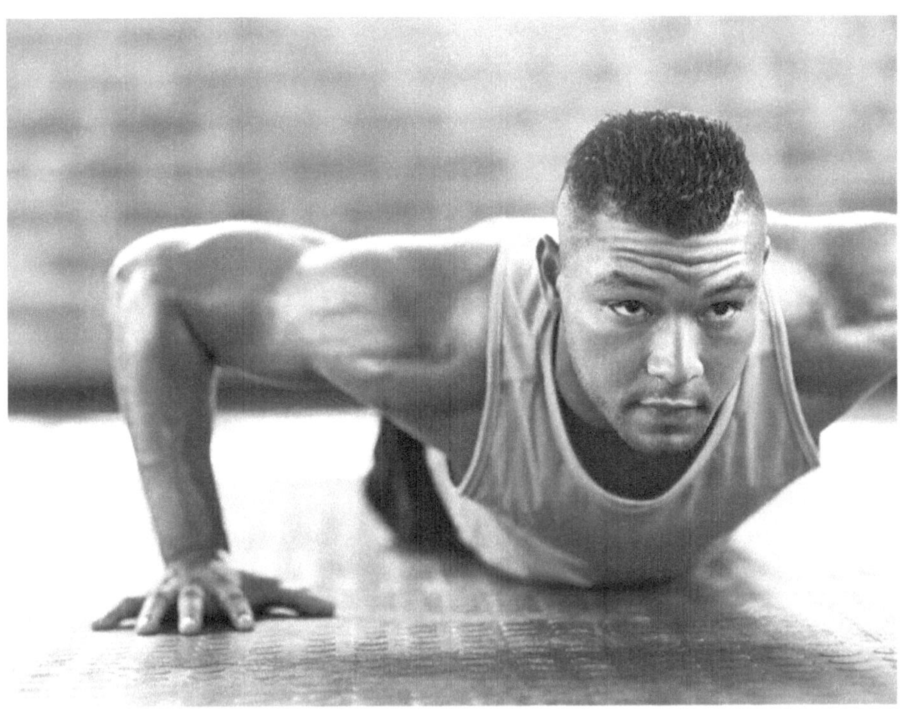

9. Bodyweight Upper Body

Directions: Repeat this circuit as many times as possible in 20 minutes.

1.   Pushups
Reps: 10

2.   Straight-leg   Situps
Reps: 10

3. Bodyweight   Triceps   Extensions
Reps: 10

4.   Plank

Duration: 30 seconds

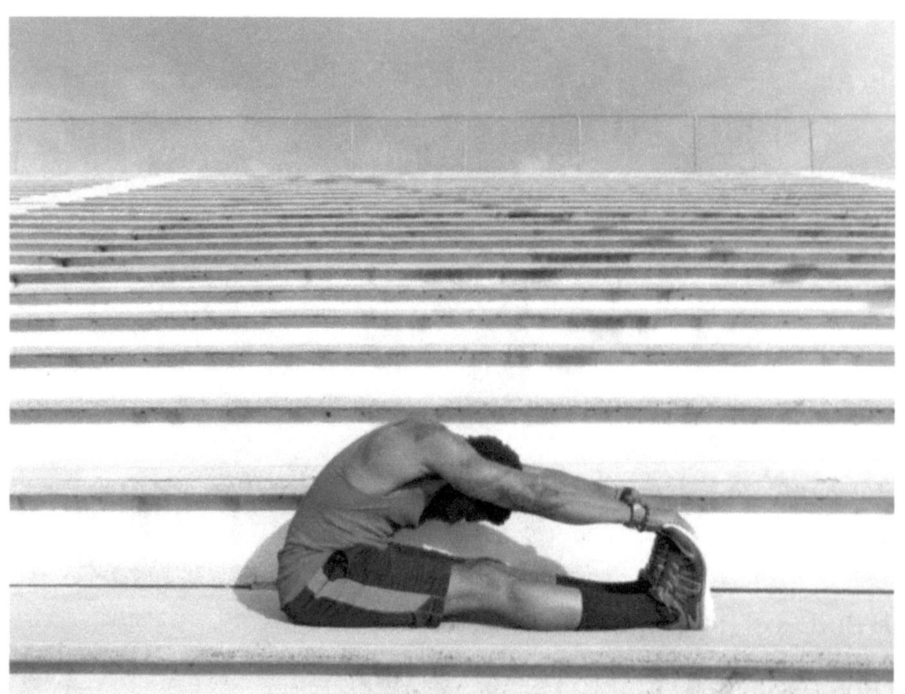

10. Bodyweight Lower Body/Abs

Directions: Do all A exercises, then all B exercises, then all C exercises.

A1.   Bulgarian   Split   Squat   Jumps
Sets: 3
Reps: 6 (each leg)

B1.   Bulgarian   Split   Squat   Countdowns
Sets: 2

Reps: 21 (6 to 1) — Do six reps, then do a six-second iso hold with your rear knee just off the floor. Go straight into five reps followed by a five-second iso hold, then four, etc, all the way down to one rep. In total, it's 21 reps, and 21 seconds of holds.

B2.	Straight-leg		Situps
Sets:			2
Reps: 15			

C1. Glute	Bridge	V	Walkouts
Sets:			2
Reps: 6			

C2.	Straight-leg	Reverse	Crunch
Sets:			2
Reps: 12			